Hearing the Person with Dementia

of related interest

Person-Centred Dementia Care
Making Services Better
Dawn Brooker
ISBN 978 1 84310 337 0
eISBN 978 1 84642 588 2

Enriched Care Planning for People with Dementia
A Good Practice Guide to Delivering Person-Centred Care
Hazel May, Paul Edwards and Dawn Brooker
ISBN 978 1 84310 405 6
eISBN 978 1 84642 960 6

Personalisation and Dementia
A Guide for Person-Centred Practice
Helen Sanderson and Gill Bailey
ISBN 978 1 84905 379 2
eISBN 978 0 85700 734 6

The Simplicity of Dementia
A Guide for Family and Carers
Huub Buijssen
ISBN 978 1 84310 321 9
eISBN 978 1 84642 096 2

Telling Tales About Dementia
Experiences of Caring
Edited by Lucy Whitman
ISBN 978 1 84310 941 9
eISBN 978 0 85700 017 0

Connecting through Music with People with Dementia
A Guide for Caregivers
Robin Rio
ISBN 978 1 84310 905 1
eISBN 978 1 84642 725 1

Puppetry in Dementia Care
Connecting through Creativity and Joy
Karrie Marshall
ISBN 978 1 84905 392 1
eISBN 978 0 85700 848 0

Activities for Older People in Care Homes
A Handbook for Successful Activity Planning
Sarah Crockett
ISBN 978 1 84905 429 4
eISBN 978 0 85700 839 8

Hearing the Person with Dementia

Person-Centred Approaches to Communication for Families and Caregivers

Bernie McCarthy

Jessica Kingsley *Publishers*
London and Philadelphia

Quote on p.48 reproduced by permission of Aitken Alexander Associates and
Edward de Bono. Copyright © Edward de Bono.
Epigraph on p.85 reproduced by permission of Habib Chaudhury.

First published in 2011
by Jessica Kingsley Publishers
73 Collier Street
London N1 9BE, UK
and
400 Market Street, Suite 400
Philadelphia, PA 19106, USA

www.jkp.com

Copyright © Bernie McCarthy 2011

Library of Congress Cataloging in Publication Data
McCarthy, Bernie.
  Hearing the person with dementia : person-centred approaches to communication for
families and caregivers / Bernie McCarthy.
    p. ; cm.
  Includes bibliographical references and index.
  ISBN 978-1-84905-186-6 (alk. paper)
  1. Dementia--Nursing. 2. Dementia--Patients--Care--Psychological aspects. 3. Dementia--
Patients--Family relationships. 4. Medical personnel and patient. I. Title.
  [DNLM: 1. Dementia--nursing. 2. Dementia--psychology. 3. Caregivers--psychology. 4.
Communication. 5. Nurse-Patient Relations. 6. Patient-Centered Care--methods. WM 220]
  RC521.M389 2011
  616.8'3--dc22
                                    2010034866

British Library Cataloguing in Publication Data
A CIP catalogue record for this book is available from the British Library

ISBN 978 1 84905 186 6
eISBN 978 0 85700 499 4

Printed and bound in Great Britain

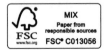

Acknowledgements

I express my gratitude to Virginia Moore and Kim Wylie for opening up the person-centred approach to seeing people who live with dementia. They have inspired me to explore and understand more deeply the meaning of being person-centred. I have also been supported by Dawn Brooker who embodies this way of being in her work and relationships and whose guidance has helped me to appreciate the more subtle aspects of helping people in organisations to be more person-centred. My life with Anne and Scarlett is the well I drink from and sit at in quiet wonderment – thank you. This book is dedicated to these people, to those who live with dementia and to those who care daily for the ones they love.

Contents

Introduction

Communication is the food of relationships. Good communication is nourishing, delightful and memorable. It creates intimacy, enriches us and we become better people. Poor communication is like bad food – poisonous and harmful.

Bernie McCarthy

Hearing the Person with Dementia is written from my experience of working to support carers of people living with dementia at home and in residential care. It is written for these carers.

Over the years that I have worked in aged care I have witnessed the powerful effect of good communication in reaching a person previously thought to be 'unreachable' because of cognitive impairment. And, sadly I have witnessed the effects of poor communication and seen the person wither before my eyes as they are misread and frustrated by care staff and/or family. I hope you will find many ideas and helpful ways of approaching interactions with the person you care for in the pages of this book. May they be happier, more contented and peacefully connected to and with us, and to their own lives, past and present.

Chapter 1

Communication

Sometimes it's a struggle

We communicate to get a message across to others, to share ideas with others and to find out what others think and feel, to build intimacy, to share and solve problems. Without the ability to communicate we struggle to maintain a sense of relationship, connection and psychological attachment to other people. This is the difficulty faced by many people with impairment in the area of communicating. They struggle to make us understand their inner experience, wants and needs, and they struggle to understand what we want of them. We struggle to understand them and get our message across to them. The struggle is fraught with frustration and, at times, tension; it can be wearing and numbing. And then there are those moments of pure joy when both seem to be thinking of the same thing, each connecting with the other person and finding understanding. It seems so easy then.

How we communicate has a profound effect on the quality of our relationships, on the quality of our lives. Whether you are a spouse or a paid carer, if you have a relationship with someone who has dementia you may be experiencing some of the difficulty of communicating with your partner, loved one or friend, or client. (For those readers working with a person with an intellectual impairment, simply change the words relating to dementia and replace them with words that match your situation. I hope this works for you.) It is not easy to maintain an equal relationship, as the dementing illness progressively affects the person's ability to contribute equally to the relationship.

The person-centred approach to communicating can keep the focus on the person and the dementing illness takes second place.

Before we go any further we need to look at how the healthy brain works and what happens when the brain is affected by dementia. In the next section we will look at the brain, how it functions and how it helps shape our experience of the world. Then there are a few questions that will test your understanding.

Dementia and the brain

The person-centred approach values all aspects of the person and this includes the biological health of the person, especially their brain. A normal brain does miraculous things to make us successful in our lives. Take a moment to think about all the decisions you have made today. You woke up, got out of bed, chose some clothes to wear, dressed yourself, ate breakfast; drove your car, walked, cycled or took public transport to work.

This marvellous brain sits in your skull cavity and is made up of billions of cells called neurons that send electrical and chemical impulses (messages) throughout the brain when sensory input comes in, and often, in response to your imagination, memory and feelings.

When your brain functions as it usually does, you can think, remember, solve problems, feel emotions, use imagination, speak and understand the speech of others, recognise objects in the world around you, and much, much more.

When the brain is affected by a disease (such as Alzheimer's) or a malfunction such as a blockage to the blood supply, or by an injury, we begin to experience life differently and may in time act differently.

If the person you care for has Alzheimer's disease the first signs you may have noticed are memory problems and some difficulty finding words. The most obvious issue about Alzheimer's is that it is progressive, i.e. the difficulties gradually become worse over time. In the early stages the person may become lost and have trouble finding their way to places that were once familiar. You will find excellent information in some detail in your Alzheimer's Association help sheets and resources from other organisations that you can find quickly in a Google search. Check the quality of what you find, as it may be written by a recognised authority, or it may not. If it is written by a university or by a recognised agency you are familiar with, you can usually trust the quality of the information.

What is most important at this point is that you stay in touch with and be sensitive to the person's feelings about what is happening to them. Each person will react in a way that makes sense to them. Or put another way, each person makes sense of the world as they perceive it to be.

This is important from the person-centred approach. Valuing the individual person's perspective helps them to maintain their social self and remain successful as a social being for as long as possible. For example, forgetting things may not be a problem emotionally to some people, but to others it may mean that they are a failure or a bad person. This may be so if they have had bad experiences of forgetting things as a child and been punished for it, as many people were. So tune into the emotional aspect of what is happening to the person when they forget, not just the obvious part (the forgetting) that you can see.

Hemispheres of the brain

There are two halves to the brain, joined in the centre, much as a cauliflower is made up of florets that are joined at the stem. Each half is believed to perform slightly different functions. One of the most important and clear differences is in language. The left hemisphere has more logical and structured thinking. The right hemisphere has more creative and expressive activity. The left hemisphere has more language function for right-handers (about 90%) than left-handers (50%).

Parietal lobe
Visuo-spatial ability
(your internal map)
Judgment of texture,
weight, size, shape
Integrates spoken and
written information

Frontal lobe
Planning
Organising
Problem-solving
Decision-making
Social awareness
Emotional control

Occipital lobe →
Visual processing
Shapes
Colours

Temporal lobe
Memory – working
and long term
Emotion
Sense experience

Cerebellum →
Balance
Muscle coordination

Lobes of the brain

There are four sections or 'lobes' we commonly talk about: frontal, parietal, occipital and temporal. Another major area is the limbic system. Brain function is a 'team' activity in which each part works with the help of other parts to produce our experience. Some areas are specialised for particular functions – for example, the temporal lobes for memory and the occipital lobes for vision. Let's look at each of the lobes.

1. Frontal lobes

Frontal lobes are just behind your forehead and are very important for shaping social behaviour (knowing how to act in the company of other people), problem-solving, abstract thinking (being able to think about ideas like 'safety' or 'morality'), ability to start and stop doing or saying things, knowing how other people feel and adjusting our behaviour to them, and making decisions. This is the 'executive', the manager that helps us control ourselves and relate with others in the world in a safe and sociable way.

The frontal lobes are not fully formed until our mid-20s, which explains why some teenagers take risks and behave in ways that frustrate and concern their parents.

The frontal lobes also help us do complex tasks, such as dressing, in the right sequence of steps.

Sarah had trouble dressing in the right order and each day walked into the dining room with her underwear over the top of her tracksuit. One day she had been to the hairdresser and walked into the dining room clearly feeling very good about herself, as you do after having your hair done, carrying her handbag and with her undies over the top of her tracksuit. The staff member came up to her and said very discreetly, 'Sarah, you've got your undies over your tracksuit'. Sarah turned around, and with hands on hips said, 'That's how we wear them here!'

2. Temporal lobes

Temporal lobes are very close by, on either side of your head in front of the ears (in the temples), and are mostly important for memory. Modern knowledge of memory is much better now than in the past. We used to talk about short-term memory, but now use the term 'working memory'. This relates to the ability to hold pieces of information in our minds long enough to do something with them, i.e. work on them. An example might be learning a phone number or making a shopping list, or remembering a person's name in a conversation so that we can use it again at the right time.

Long-term memory, on the other hand, is the ability we have to store information/experiences/ knowledge for long periods – up to a lifetime. We can usually do this by repeating the information often until it is 'learned'. Then we can retrieve it again when, for example, someone says, 'Where were you born?'

Another important type of memory is 'semantic'. This is the ability to remember what things mean. Knowing what the written word 'carrot' means or what a picture of a 'shirt' or 'toilet' indicates is very important for your basic ability to function in areas of life such as cooking, dressing or toileting.

3. Parietal lobes

The next brain area is the parietal lobes. This is the area responsible for your ability to find your way and not get lost, for example remembering where the freezer is located in the supermarket, or your car in the car park on the way out. It also helps put together the parts of a situation into a whole impression, for example combine all the sensory stimuli of a football match into 'an experience' of the match; or organise words into a pattern such as a sentence that conveys an idea. It also helps you recognise objects such as clothing or food. It helps us complete calculations.

4. Occipital lobes

Finally the occipital lobe, located at the back of your head, is where vision is processed. Here the brain interprets what you see (so you could say you do have eyes in the back of your head!). Vision can decrease for people who have brain impairment as the brain cells may be lost in the progress of the disease. Therefore brightness and even lighting, absence of glare, and contrasts between objects and their background become much more important for the person to function indoors.

Limbic system and emotion

The final major feature of the brain for our discussion of communication is the limbic system. This area is important for emotional experience, which is central to good communication. It consists of areas of all the lobes and surrounds the 'reptilian' or ancient area of our brain that we have in common with other vertebrates. The limbic system helps us put an 'emotional tag' on all our experiences. (We like it or don't like it. We feel attracted to some people and not others. We had a good time or we were afraid or angry.)

Emotions are a vital part of human living, as the feelings we have help us to appreciate, value and love the people, roles, activities and interactions we have with each other. Without them we have only survival reactions to guide our choices. Life would become mundane and lacking in colour without our emotions.

The limbic system helps us to sort out our preferences and make choices based on feelings, and often on memories of past experiences that may have been pleasant and enjoyable or fearful and unpleasant. In trauma, this system helps protect us from extremely unpleasant emotional experiences by sometimes 'blocking off' feelings from the sensory parts of what we experienced in the past. For the person with dementia, past trauma can interfere with current day-to-day life because it can be confused with what is happening now. The limbic system recognises the feeling similar to what we experienced in the past, and memories may surface that have nothing to do with now, but a lot to do with what happened a long time ago, when it felt similar to how it feels right now.

Tom fought in World War II in Borneo and was taken prisoner by the Japanese. He was interned in a camp for several years, during which time he experienced severe hardship and suffering, and witnessed atrocities that have stayed with him in memories. Now in his 80s, with dementia for the past few years, he sleeps poorly and wakes in a sweat at night with nightmares he can't explain. He becomes angry and blaming of staff when they ask him to do something like go to the toilet. He doesn't like feeling dominated or made to do things now. His body is thin and wasted, like it was when he was a prisoner. He feels afraid and believes he is back in the past.

Tom's mind and body are re-experiencing the wartime distress he endured, because both his mind and his body 'feel' as they did then.

The brain in daily functioning

Let us look now at several functions the brain helps us with through the day.

Memory

The brain is particularly good at helping us work out whether we have seen things before or not. If we see something new, our brain focuses on it and tries to check if it is important. For instance, if we are passing hundreds of cars on the way to work, our brain does not attend to each one. However, if one car hits our car we will remember the colour or make of the car because it has become important or significant for us. This tells us something about how we remember. If something is significant, it is easier to remember. Also, if it is emotionally important (like a car that hit us), we will remember it.

This is why a person with dementia may remember some things and not others. They will remember a staff member whom they like or dislike, but may not remember others towards whom they have no reaction or feeling.

The other important factor about memory is repetition. We learn by repeating things over and over, and so they become more easy to recall. This is important for people with dementia, who can continue to learn new information if we repeat it over again to them within the span of their decreasing working memory. You may be able to use this to assist the person with dementia to maintain their connection with past experiences. This is simply reminiscence and is incredibly valuable as a means of helping the person stay in touch with their identity.

Language

Speaking our thoughts in a form that others can understand is a basic human ability and we often take it for granted. The complement of this ability is comprehension or understanding of what others say to us. This two-way ability is fundamental to human socialising and facilitates intimacy, problem-solving, diplomacy and the communication of everyday needs and wants.

In Alzheimer's disease it gradually becomes more difficult for the person to find the right words. As well as memory loss, the person can have increasing difficulty in participating in a conversation with the ease and fluency they may have once had.

Dennis was a successful journalist who prided himself on his extensive vocabulary and command of the English language. When he began having difficulty finding the right word, and making mistakes he would never previously have made, he began to lose confidence and he stopped writing. He withdrew and stayed at home out of embarrassment that he could no longer think and speak with the once rich skill he had prided himself on.

The senses and the brain

The brain helps us understand what is happening in the world around us. It does this by taking in information from all the senses – vision, hearing, touch, taste and smell. These channels of information flow into the brain with such speed that it has evolved a way to focus only on the information that is changing and concentrate on this, while processing the other information automatically, so that we don't have to concentrate on it. This ability frees up our brain to focus only on the parts of our life that are changing and not its routine, familiar aspects.

> Jean was a florist who knew flowers and plants so well that she could assemble a beautiful arrangement without having to spend much time on it. She did it automatically. But now that she has dementia she has trouble doing the everyday things she once found effortless, and when asked to do the once familiar and enjoyable task of arranging a vase of flowers, she becomes upset and overwhelmed.

Bodily sensations

Our bodies are connected to our brains by neurons that stimulate muscles and receive information from our skin and muscles. A hotplate on a stove can be hot to the touch, and our brains sense this and instruct our muscles to pull away to protect us from harm.

Our brains can read what is happening in our bodies too. The inner sensation you have when you are hungry, thirsty or need to go to the toilet alerts you to whatever action you need to take to solve the problem of how you feel in your body.

Mavis was very particular about her personal hygiene and always left plenty of time to go to the toilet wherever she travelled. She would plan trips around toilet stops and always 'went' before she left the house. Now that her brain is not reading her interior sensation of a full bladder, she is often agitated by the feeling and not able to work out what to do about it. Recently she had an accident or two that distressed her very much, with some embarrassment about making such a very personal mistake. She now gets anxious and refuses to go out on the bus or for walks in the morning.

Pain and the brain

The experience of pain is complex. The brain senses that a part of the body is in distress and interprets this sensation, causing the body to react to the sensation. For the person with dementia, recognising that a sensation is about pain may be difficult. They may be unaware they are in pain, or unable to problem-solve about the uncomfortable and distressing experience they are having. The idea that it is pain may not occur to them. As a result they may be unable to do anything helpful about it, either by telling someone else about it (which is what we do most of the time) to get help, or by doing something about it themselves. To act successfully about pain requires a complex sequence of thoughts that connect up, resulting in relief from the pain, and this may be too much to expect of a person with dementia.

For us the important issue here is to be able to recognise the signs of pain that a person with dementia may communicate using nonverbal 'language'. Remember that behaviour is a language. Pain can be communicated through facial expression, posture, favouring a body part, vocalising (making noises or sounds), changes in behaviour or mood. Look for the signs and you may pick it up more quickly than the person with dementia, and be able to provide appropriate relief.

Tiredness

The person who lives with dementia may not be able to tell you they are tired and need to go to bed. As with other sensations, the experience of tiredness requires an ability to detect, understand and then act to address the problem. The person may not be able to do this successfully. What we see is the person becoming more agitated, irritable, restless or confused, perhaps. Each individual will be unique in their response to tiredness, so we need to get to know a person's way of acting when they are tired, and adopt an approach that helps them to remedy the problem without making them feel overwhelmed or dominated. This leads us into the person-centred way of communicating that helps us to focus our attention on the well-being of the person, and not just on the outcome of fulfilling tasks that have traditionally been seen as the purpose of caregiving.

Infections and the brain

In an older person an infection can cause the brain to malfunction more severely than in a younger person. Such infections might include urinary tract infections

(UTIs), chest and upper respiratory infections, or wounds that are not healing well.

The physical health of the people we care for is as important to us as carers as their emotional health. Therefore it is important to obtain medical diagnosis and treatment quickly and effectively for the person with dementia. Sometimes leaving it for several days before obtaining medical help can result in a poor outcome for the person, as their ability to fight infection can be lower than that of a younger person.

The brain and food

We know a good diet is vital for muscle strength and bone density. Your brain also relies on the nutrients that you consume in food and fluid to be able to do all the thinking, remembering, feeling, sensing and perceiving that you take for granted every day. A good diet is vital for a person living with dementia, just as it is for us all. Poor food equals poor brain function. Good food equals better brain function. So a balanced diet will enhance memory and thinking, help the person to be in a good mood and assist them to function to their full capacity. There is a great deal of knowledge available about balanced nutrition. If you are caring in the home and you are in doubt, consult a dietician or nutritionist to design for you and the person you care for a diet suitable for each of you in terms of age, physical condition and lifestyle.

Exercise 1.1

Brain functions in everyday life

1. What area of the brain is responsible for social behaviour?

2. What abilities are impaired early in the progress of Alzheimer's disease?

3. How does the limbic system help us function?

4. What areas of Tom's brain are involved in causing him to react strongly with emotion now? (See page 19.)

5. If you had problems with speech, what area(s) of the brain might be affected?

6. What parts of your brain do you use when you are getting dressed in the morning?

7. What areas of the brain are not working for Sarah? (See page 16.)

8. How does the limbic system help us react to the world around us?

9. Is the limbic system a reliable source of information about our current experience or does it confuse past and present?

10. How does your diet affect the way your brain functions?

11. How does your diet affect your mood?

Chapter 2

Hearing the Person – VIPS

Now that we have considered the brain and its function we will go into more depth looking at the person-centred approach to being with a person with dementia.

Person-centredness has become a common focus in modern health care. It is a term used to mean many things, and so can in the end mean nothing at all. We need a simple model or way of understanding this term. The simplest and yet most comprehensive approach is the 'VIPS' model (Brooker 2004, 2007).

The VIPS approach, developed by Dawn Brooker of the University of Worcester, consists of four elements, represented by the letters of the common acronym for 'very important persons' – VIPS:

V = value
I   = individualised
P = perspective
S = social

These four key elements provide a simple yet sophisticated approach to understanding and using person-centred communication.

- Every person living with dementia has enduring *value* that the illness or impairment cannot destroy. So no matter what impairments the person has, they are still a person.

- *Individualised* refers to the need to adapt all we do and say (and all we don't do or say) to the particular person we have in front of us, and to avoid using a one-size-fits-all approach to communicating and to the way we behave.

- *Perspective* is the perspective of the person with dementia, i.e., what do they think, feel, touch, taste, smell, hear, see, want, need and remember?

- *Social* is the recognition that we are 'social beings' in need of connection/intimacy/bonding with others in a social setting of relationship, family, group, tribe, town and nation. It is in this social dimension that our personal value can be diminished or enhanced by the way other people relate with us. Socially we need to be respected, to trust others and to engage in the mainstream of life, so that we can feel OK about ourselves. These are fundamental human needs, to trust and be respected (we'll talk more about these needs later).

VIPS: Value

Dementia challenges our view of the value of every person. The condition changes the way people function and behave in everyday life, and this has traditionally caused society to regard people with dementia as being less than human. This uncomfortable thought has shaped the way we care for people with dementia up to modern times. However, the person-centred approach regards the person as having intrinsic value.

All people have unique and everlasting value that cannot be taken from them, no matter how impaired or disabled they become. The value of a person is not dependent on their ability to communicate, think, problem-solve or contribute productively to society. It is not related to social status. Each person is important, regardless of their social standing or wealth.

All very well in theory, you might say. But I need to feel beautiful to feel OK about myself. I need praise or positive strokes to feel good about myself. Or I need to contribute with my work or be successful to feel good about myself. And indeed I feel bad about myself when I am treated badly by others or act badly toward others. So what do these experiences have to do with a theoretical value I have, even though I may not actually feel that I have any value? To help us understand this we must look at personhood.

Value and personhood

Personhood is our subjective sense of who we are as a person in relationship with other people and the world around us, and shapes our thinking, feelings and behaviour in relation to others. The late Professor Tom Kitwood from the United Kingdom described personhood as:

> the standing or status bestowed on one human being by others, in the context of human relationship and

social being. It implies recognition, respect and trust. (Kitwood 1997, p.8)

We are persons because we are in relationship with others. We are always in relationship with others, whether that is another person or group or (in a religious or spiritual belief system) in relationship with God. We are constituted as a person by being in relationship. This makes us the unique persons we are. The quality of those relationships shapes our own personhood. Our personhood is dynamic and always changing. It is responsive to people, situations and events.

We are not born with a sense of personhood. Our sense of personhood emerges and changes throughout our lives as our sense of self is shaped by the way other people treat us, our responses to situations and the meaning these experiences have for us. This is especially true of our attachment figures from infancy (usually our mother and father) who help us create a sense of trust in the world, if their love is consistently available and gives us a sense of safety and affection. As we grow up, if people communicate with us in a way that is demeaning, or ignore us, or criticise us unreasonably or bully us, our self-esteem might decrease. If it happens often enough, for long enough, you might begin to believe negative thoughts about yourself. You may begin to feel like a 'non-person'. In this way, your sense of personhood can be diminished.

On the other hand, if people treat us with respect, listen attentively and validate our feelings, respect our perspective, include us in decisions, offer choices and bother to get to know and understand us, our self-esteem can be enhanced and we feel good about ourselves. This enhances our personhood.

Long-term maltreatment or trauma can shape a person's sense of themselves in a lasting manner. There is some evidence to suggest that our basic personality is set by early adulthood and does not change remarkably after that. On the other hand, some suggest that a sense of self is set by the age of seven years.

A way of thinking about this is in terms of a tree. There are different types of trees: oak, beech, eucalyptus and pine. Each grows according to its nature. Then come soil, wind and rain to shape the tree's growth in particular ways. The soil, wind and rain are like the changing social environment that surrounds us as we grow. Over time the tree is shaped by these factors and grows in a certain direction, may become stunted or grows vigorously, all shaped by the environment in which it grows. So, too, we develop and are influenced by the social relationships we are born into and experience as we grow into childhood, adolescence and adulthood. The moment-to-moment changes in the way people treat us have an effect on our personhood, which we bring into each situation, and diminish or enhance it just as lack of water and nutrients can cause a tree to eventually wither and die, but rain and good soil enhance its growth and it flourishes.

If a person has a cognitive impairment, personhood is more easily diminished by the way others communicate with them. You and I are able to walk away from unpleasant behaviour and communication. The person with dementia may not be able to walk away, or find the words to say, or assert themselves socially or solve the problem they are faced with. This can result in diminished self-esteem and making less effort to involve themselves in social situations. The person with a cognitive impairment may withdraw, not contribute, avoid going to gatherings and cease to initiate social contact. The more they do this, the more they will lose their verbal skills, as social withdrawal causes the advancing dementia to rob the person of their remaining abilities more quickly. We know from research that social engagement is associated with increases in brain volume. So, too, social withdrawal can result in decreased brain volume as the disease progresses.

As time passes the person may develop low mood and feel less confident about themselves, eventually moving into depression. We know from research that people who become depressed generally have more medical issues, attend the doctor more and live shorter lives than people who are not depressed.

How we communicate with a person with a cognitive impairment has significant social and physical health consequences. If the social environment is positive and inclusive, offering everyone the opportunity to contribute to conversation in a socially equal way, the person with a cognitive impairment may find they are relaxed and feel accepted. They can then use their skills, and maintain their roles and status as a normal part of the family or other group. So, cognitive impairment notwithstanding sensitive communication can maintain the person in the social group for longer, and maintain their personhood and skills for longer in the face of the advancing disease.

We can slow the effect of progressing dementia by using consistently sensitive, thoughtful and inclusive communication. We can improve the health of the people we care for by communicating with them in a person-centred manner.

Sarah has been ostracised after wearing her undies over her tracksuit when she came into the dining room. The other ladies will not speak to her and ignore her when she comes to join in activities. One or two have loudly told her to go away. Sarah has lost confidence and wants to stay in her room. She sits and looks lost for long periods. She sleeps a lot more now. One of the staff has made an effort to go to her room and visit her each morning to talk and reminisce with her. Slowly Sarah has connected and begun to trust this carer and has agreed to go shopping with her. They make sure all is right with her clothes and they have a very happy time. Sarah is a different person after the trip and makes good eye contact with staff and smiles when people go up to her. Staff are more careful to make sure she is dressed successfully and help her avoid the social problems her dressing mistake has caused.

Value and well-being

We have been discussing the positive and negative impact of communication on the personhood of the person we care for and about. Another way to understand this is in terms of well-being. Communication affects well-being.

Well-being is that quality of life we experience when we feel good about ourselves, others and our world. Signs of well-being include: positive mood, assertiveness, relaxed body, humour, taking social initiative, engagement with the world around us, taking pleasure, being helpful, being affectionate, having self-respect, creative self-expression and sensitivity to the emotional needs of others (Bradford Dementia Group 2005).

Value and ill-being

The other side of the well-being coin is ill-being. As we mentioned earlier, when communication is negative and relationships are not healthy, the effect on the person with a cognitive impairment can be profound and much more dramatic than the negative effect on you and me.

Ill-being is the negative experience of existence, other people and our world. It can be seen in negative mood, feeling depressed or despairing, unresolved grieving over losses, intense anger, listlessness, apathy or withdrawal, agitation, restlessness, physical illness or pain, bodily tension, being easily 'walked over' and showing anxiety, fear or boredom (Bradford Dementia Group 2005).

Example

- Words that signal well-being: I feel...

    pleased, happy, loved, good, appreciated, valued, connected, close, special, elated.

- Words that signal ill-being: I feel...

    angry, sad, frustrated, annoyed, alone, lonely, isolated, useless, suspicious, used, betrayed, depressed, anxious, worried.

Communicating well with people with dementia and other forms of cognitive impairment is crucial for their continued well-being – physical, emotional, social and spiritual. Just performing the technical aspects of communication well is not enough. It is easy to know that we should use short sentences or pause between instructions. To be able to bring yourself (your personhood) into the interaction, and maintain an awareness of the personhood of the other person, requires more than technical expertise and knowledge. It is an art that calls on your personal involvement, personal presence and awareness of the emotional and psychological effects of your behaviour on the other person and the consequences for their well-being. It requires you to practise being focused on the welfare of another person, with the aim of sustaining or enhancing the personhood of that person regardless of their disability or attractiveness to us.

Exercise 2.1

VIPS – Value: personhood, well-being and ill-being

1. What values are important in your life? To help you focus on this question, think about what you choose to do with your money and your time. That will show you what you value.

2. How do you see people who have impairments of body or mind?

3. What affects your personhood?

4. How do you need to be treated by others to feel good about yourself?

5. What behaviour from others causes you to feel bad about yourself?

6. How important is it for you to be focused on the well-being of another person?

VIPS: Individual

As noted previously, good communication requires an ability to adapt your words and approach to the particular person in front of you. The 'old culture of dementia care' (Kitwood 1997) used a 'one-size-fits-all' approach in which the person disappeared and we only saw the disease or problems. This institutional approach disregarded the uniqueness of each person and used the same approach for everyone.

This 'one-size-fits-all' approach to people living with dementia means that you apply the same rules and routines in the same way to everyone, without flexibility. This approach is simple and does not require much thought or decision-making and is easier for some people to use. But it often leads to diminished personhood, lower levels of well-being and higher levels of ill-being. It is harmful to the person, toxic. It is often the reason why we get aggressive responses from people.

Johanna was a quiet lady who lived a busy life of helping others in her volunteer work. She had always prized the respect she gave to others and valued the way others treated her. She liked being recognised and respected when she walked in the shopping centre and her neighbourhood. When she was admitted to the nursing home with dementia she began to react strongly when carers commenced showering or toileting. They called her 'Jo' and 'Darling' and they didn't really give her a choice about the shower or when to go to the toilet. She lashed out with her fists and cried loudly to 'get away from me'. Johanna was feeling angry, furious at the lack of respect she felt from the carers who approached her.

Johanna's distress is a good example of the need for carers to tailor their actions to the individual needs of the person they are caring for. We must adapt our approach to be flexible when responding to the person we have in front of us, rather than relate as if the person is an 'object', as if the person doesn't really exist. Just because a friend or colleague said something in a certain way, or used a particular strategy to solve a problem, doesn't mean it is suitable for the person *you* are caring for. You must adapt your approach to the person in front of you.

Imagine if you were treated in the following way. You visit the dentist for your regular dental check-up and he/she begins filling your perfectly healthy back teeth, because this is what worked with the previous patient, whose back teeth were decayed. You would think you had visited a crazy person. You'd be out of that chair before you could say 'malpractice'! The tragic aspect of this example is that the person with dementia that you are caring for may not be able to voice their need or will. Sometimes they cannot even voice their disapproval. You are all they have at that moment, so your actions, your words and your attitude need to be purposeful, respectful and kind, and appropriate to the person you have in front of you.

So how do we do this? We get to know the person's life-story as well as we can. If the person you are caring for is your husband or wife and you know them very well, you have a head start. (However, this very familiarity can sometimes lead to biased relating that may not be helpful in the current situation!)

If you do not have a personal relationship with the person you will need to get to know them from scratch. All being well, the policy at your workplace will be to document a detailed life-story gathered from people such as family members or friends (or the person with dementia themselves). Read this story and become familiar with the person's preferences, likes and dislikes, emotional dispositions, moods and past patterns of communication. Look for anything that tells you, 'Maybe they would feel good about themselves if *I* did this…or if *they* did this…'

If you are unable to find out much about the person from others (and unfortunately this is often the case in modern society), you will need to compile a profile of their wants, desires, needs, emotional dispositions or tendencies, moods and patterns of communication, from your own observations (and those of your colleagues). Note down all information you can glean from your activity of daily living (ADL) interactions, their engagement in activities and lifestyle actions, food preferences, and stories they tell you when, for example, you are helping them prepare for bed. You will pick up small pieces of information as you care for the person. It is tempting to see these as unimportant. However, they can form the basis of images to give those who care for this person a sense of who they are and have been. All information is valuable. Don't go home at the end of your shift with it in your head. Write it down so that others can take advantage of it too.

The best way to write about the person's life is in a 'story'. While you may start out with a checklist of information as you gather it, at some point put the information into a story. Each point you note about the person can become a sentence that fills out their preferences.

Example

[List format]

- likes marshmallow
- dislikes porridge

[Narrative/story format]

Tom likes marshmallows toasted over a fire because he had these when he was a Boy Scout in the country. Marshmallows remind him of his youth and the great times he had in the Scouts.

Tom dislikes porridge because he had it every morning at his grandmother's house where he stayed for the years when his mother was ill.

By including the significance of the like/dislike, that is, what it means for the person, you can create an opportunity for well-being with a gentle reminiscence prompt about the marshmallows and toasting them over fires, such as, 'Tom, you were a Boy Scout, weren't you?' or 'Tom, when you were in the Scouts, did you toast marshmallows in the campfire?' Or you could use a simple statement without the question: 'Tom, you were in the Boy Scouts. You enjoyed toasting marshmallows over the fire.' The person feels pleased at the memory you have helped to stimulate, and settled and peaceful because at some level it feels familiar. It can be as simple as that.

The narrative format is more dignified and respectful, as well as easier to read and engage with. We like telling and listening to stories, and if you can tell a tale about the person you will find that other people will read it and digest the information more readily than they would from a long list.

What information should you include in your life-story? There are many models to choose from and no one right way to do it. If you go to the internet you will find some examples of life-story work in the care of older people, and many are in a format accessible and ready to use.

If you are looking for a model that is focused on building a rich story that can be used to enhance a person-centred approach, you may wish to select from the menu of options below. Remember that you will need to select the headings that are relevant to the person you are caring for. Try to avoid the trap of using a one-size-fits-all approach! Using the entire list of headings will be overwhelming for some people. Select what you need for the person you are with. You may have some of this information already from other sources, so omit unnecessary questions.

Remember to record feelings expressed by the person when they answer the question. This will give you a clue as to whether this is likely to create ill-being or well-being for them if you revisit this topic in the future. For example, Tom was uncomfortable remembering his mother's illness. Using these words, we create a picture or map of the person's emotional memory landscape.

LIFE-STORY PROFILING

1. **Birth**
   a. Place of birth.
   b. Date of birth.
   c. Conditions of birth.
   d. Any stories relating to birth.
   e. Significance of the name you were given.

2. **Family of origin**
   a. Parents
      i. Who are they?
      ii. Dates of birth, marriage, death.
      iii. Where born, married, died?
      iv. How did they die?
      v. Who were you close to, not close to?
         Which parent are you more similar to?
         What makes you similar to this parent?
   b. Siblings
      i. Who were they in birth order?
      ii. Have any of your siblings died?
   c. What was life like at home during your
      childhood? Happy home? Sad home? Stressed
      home?
   d. What stories do your siblings tell about life at
      home during your childhood years?

3. **Locations**
   a. Where did you live and when? Why did you live
      there?
   b. Did you grow up on a farm? If so, where? What
      did you farm?
   c. Which places did you like most? What did you
      like about these places?

    d.   Which places did you dislike most? What did you dislike about these places?

    e.   Describe some of the places in detail if you can.

4. **Childhood illnesses**
   a. What illnesses can you remember from childhood?
   b. What illnesses did other family members have during their childhood years?
   c. Were parents ill at any time?

5. **Parental work**
   a. What work did mother and/or father do?
   b. Were mother or father absent for periods of time due to work? What was this like?
   c. Did they tell you much about their work?
   d. Did you have to work with them during your growing up years? What did you have to do? Did your siblings also have to do this?

6. **Parental discipline**
   a. How did your parents discipline you and your siblings?
   b. Which of your parents was the one who did this mostly?
   c. What things were said to discipline you?
   d. How did you feel about their discipline at the time?
   e. How do you feel about their discipline now?

7. **School**
   a. Where did you go to school?
   b. How old were you when you began school?
   c. How far from home was your school? (If more than one write details for each.)
   d. What did you like best about school? What did you like least?
   e. What was your best subject at school?

  f. Did you like sport at school?

  g. Which team/house were you a member of at school?

  h. Which teachers do you remember? What makes them memorable?

  i. What friends did you have at school? Did any of these people remain friends into your adult years?

  j. Did you hold any positions while at school such as prefect, house captain, student council member? (List others as appropriate to your country.)

  k. What school projects are memorable?

  l. How old were you when you left school? For what reason did you leave school?

8. Further study

  a. What further study have you done? Where did you study?

  b. Did you choose this study or was it chosen for you?

  c. What subjects did you enjoy most?

  d. What friends did you make during this time?

  e. What did you do to socialise?

9. Recreation

  a. What did your family do to relax?

  b. Did you play sport at school or on weekends? What sports?

  c. What were you good at in sports?

  d. What was your best sporting achievement?

  e. What is your most memorable experience in sport?

10. Driving

  a. When did you get your driver's licence? Where? What were the circumstances?

b. What was your first car?

c. What cars have you had since? Which ones have you liked the most?

d. Did you have any car accidents in your driving career? Were you injured?

11. Employment

a. How old were you when you commenced your first job?

b. Did you have holiday employment? What jobs did you do? Did you like them?

12. Wartime – armed forces

a. Have you been involved in a war? Which wars have you been involved with?

b. Did you serve in the armed forces? Which country did you serve? (If no, go to Question 13.)

c. What was your highest rank? What company did you belong to?

d. What theatres of war did you serve in?

e. Tell me about the wartime experiences that have shaped your life since.

f. What was it like coming home?

g. How do you think the war has affected your life?

h. Have you had any nightmares, flashbacks or difficulty talking about the war? Have you found you would rather avoid anything to do with the war?

13. Wartime – for those who did not serve in the armed forces

a. What did you do during the war?

b. What was life like during the war?

c. What was the most difficult thing about wartime?

    d.   Did anyone you know die during the war?

    e.   What was it like after the war when the soldiers came home?

    f.   Have you had any nightmares, flashbacks or difficulty talking about the war? Have you found you would rather avoid anything to do with the war?

    g.   Did you stay in touch with friends made during the war?

14. Films

    a.   Did you go to the picture theatre when you were young?

    b.   Whom did you go with?

    c.   What films did you see?

    d.   What news clips do you remember from those times?

    e.   What films have you seen in more recent years that stay in your mind?

    f.   What film stars did you like most? Male? Female?

    g.   What type of films do you like most?

15. Songs/music

    a.   Do you like music? What sort? Jazz, pop, country and western, rock, war songs, classical?

    b.   Do you have a favourite composer/songwriter?

    c.   Do you like listening to music all the time? If no, what times do you enjoy listening to music?

    d.   What music do you like to relax with?

    e.   Did you play any musical instruments?

    f.   If so, who taught you?

    g.   Was music important in your family?

16. **Cooking**
    a. Do you know how to cook?
    b. What are you best at cooking?
    c. What is your favourite recipe/food?
    d. Who taught you to cook?
    e. Did you learn to cook for fun or because you had to?
    f. What was it like in your mother's kitchen when you were little and she was cooking? Did she let you lick the spoon?
    g. Do you like to cook these days?

17. **Machinery**
    a. What machines did you have at your place when you were young?

18. **Clubs/groups**
    a. What groups did you belong to throughout your life?
    b. What did you enjoy most about these groups?

19. **Travel/holidays**
    a. Did you travel outside [your own country]? Where to? What countries did you like the most?
    b. What did you do on your holidays overseas?
    c. Who did you travel with?
    d. Where did you go for holidays as a family?
    e. What sort of things did you do?

20. **Hobbies**
    a. What did you spend your time doing when you were not at work?
    b. What did you enjoy most about this activity?

Remembering

> Memory is a way of holding onto the things you love, the things you are, the things you never want to lose.

> *From the television show* The Wonder Years

> A memory is what is left when something happens and does not completely unhappen.

> *Edward de Bono*

Memories are our way of being in touch with our past and future in the present moment. We stand on a timeline that stretches into our past and the other way into our future. We have a sense of who we are, our identity, in remembering all the events, people and feelings that have made us who we are. We confirm this sense of self by remembering. Reminiscence is a useful way to help people whose memory is not working as it should to stay in touch with their identity, their story, their self.

This can happen in the everyday interactions we engage in, if we have the sensitivity to remember to include the whole of the person in our interaction with them, and not just focus on completing the task we have before us. Keep the whole person in the forefront of your mind. This includes as much as you can know of them.

We are the bearers of their life-story. In as much as they have told you or someone else has told you about them, their lives have become part of your memories of life now. They are part of you and you carry their life within you, in your thoughts and memories of them.

Exercise 2.2

VIPS – Individual

1. What makes you a unique person?

2. What important facts does someone need to know about you if they are to treat you with respect?

3. Write down your routine in the morning so that a person who does not know you could take you through that same routine in a way that makes you feel comfortable and understood.

4. How would you write that story for the person you care for? Perhaps you could make a start.

VIPS: Perspective

The person-centred approach to care involves taking the perspective of the other person we are communicating with – that is, communicating on their terms, as they see the world, not on our terms or perspective of the world. If the person has a cognitive impairment, their perspective will be at times more difficult to get in touch with. It is no less important. In fact it is much *more* important, as the person may be unable to communicate their perspective without our assistance and understanding.

Traditionally, the person with dementia was assumed not to have a perspective on the world, or if they did, it was assumed that they were unable to communicate it and could not be understood. So we didn't bother. We acted as if they were mindless, thoughtless and emotionless.

Now, contemporary care of people living with dementia recognises that they do indeed have an active and dynamic perspective on the world. They have a view and feelings about the people around them. They like and dislike what we do, how we act, what we say. If you listen quietly to people sitting in a residential facility lounge room and you wait till the staff have left the room, you will hear them make comments about the staff and the activity they have been asked to participate in. 'I don't want to do knitting.' 'She is a boss.' 'She's nice.' Or, as a friend related her experience once to me, when the nurses left the room, the ladies sitting together in the lounge were highly amused when one of them stated, 'Don't they all have big bums?!'

What many people fail to realise is that in reality, our behaviour is an act of communication. Accordingly, people living with dementia communicate their perspective to us with their actions. How the person with dementia acts tells us what they want, like, or do dislike and not want. This is the language of behaviour, of the spoken and unspoken. (I am indebted to Virginia Moore, who is the Manager of Customer Well-being for the Brightwater Care Group and brought Dementia Care Mapping to Australia, for this very apt description of the meaning of the actions of a person living with dementia.) If we can understand and speak this language we will be able to respond accurately to the person's communication to us.

So how should our communication be if we are to take this perspective seriously? We need to ask ourselves what our beliefs are about this perspective. Do we believe that people with dementia do indeed have a take on the world, others and themselves? If so, how do we need to change the way we communicate? May I suggest that listening is the starting point? Really listening. And not just to the words. Listening for the meaning, the same way we do with people who do not have dementia. Listening for the emotional messages and to the language of the body. What needs are being communicated by the person? What are they telling us? The following five psychological needs were identified by Professor Tom Kitwood and Kathleen Bredin in the late 1980s (Kitwood and Bredin 1992):

1. *Comfort*: The need for comfort can be felt physically, emotionally or socially. Comfort is the human experience of satisfaction of a need that gives us pleasure or release from pain and distress. A massage may be comforting. So too may a good meal, particularly if it reminds us of a past meal with friends or family. Remembering bygone pleasant events can be comforting, as such reminiscence connects us with our life-story and meaningful past experiences that affirm our identity.

2. *Attachment*: The need to be attached to other people/objects/places is a fundamental human experience that begins in the womb. It concerns our desire for food, safety and affection, and is sustained in our relationships with others throughout our lives. (We will explore this more fully in the next section on the social dimension.)

3. *Identity*: We need to know who we are, to have an identity. Who are you? How do you know you

are you? The answer to these questions is our sense of personal identity that grows with us as we develop and accumulate life experiences and memories and plans for the future.

We define ourselves, our self-image and self-esteem, by being in relationship with the physical world, with other people and with ourselves. Other people treat us well and build our self-esteem, or treat us poorly and damage our self-esteem. In this way our identity is enhanced or damaged by our relationships with others.

4. *Inclusion*: Inclusion is our need to be part of the group we belong to. Think of the groups you belong to. They are many and varied and might include the family, neighbourhood, school, workplace or clubs. You may be part of friendship groups that have no particular membership but keep changing.

We need to be recognised, to have our personhood valued by another person and by being included in social life. Being ignored is damaging to our sense of self, our personhood. Yet this is what often happens to people living with dementia, not out of a deliberate intention to cause harm, but simply because conversations move too quickly.

Listen to your conversations and notice how quickly they move and change direction and topic. This requires good short-term memory to stay connected to the topics and keep up with the flow of ideas. The person with dementia may not be able to contribute to a conversation as quickly or as fluently as we do and so they can be left behind. As often happens at parties, the conversation moves on and we stand there, silent and excluded, until the moment arrives when we can join in again. For the person with dementia, keeping the thread of the conversation in mind may be too much to ask of their memory, and they fall out of the social interaction and into social isolation very quickly. This damages their sense of inclusion, their sense of identity and their confidence.

5. *Occupation*: We all need to be able to do something in life. Sitting idle might be attractive for a few days, but after a while we become bored and distracted. If this continues we can shift into a depressed mood and outlook.

Occupation is important for our personhood. We need to be effective and productive in the world around us. We build, create, love, sing, think and laugh. In so many ways we occupy ourselves. The word 'engagement' describes our *connection* with the world around us. We engage with tasks and people in ways that draw us out of ourselves and into relationship and productivity. This engagement enhances our personhood.

The person with dementia may be unable to sustain their own engagement due to memory loss or poor concentration, despite being interested and motivated. Even motivation can be a problem at times. Some people living with dementia may be unmotivated, and this can be due to malfunctioning of the frontal lobes of the brain where our ability to start and stop behaviour is located. The brain doesn't 'start' the person, and so they sit, unless we cause them to start doing something. This can be seen most clearly in eating, when a person may sit with a meal in front of them and not take up the fork to commence eating unless prompted to by another person.

Exercise 2.3

VIPS – Perspective

1. What are the five core psychological needs and how are they present in your life? How do you act when they are not met?

2. What makes your perspective so unique and different from those around you?

3. What gives you comfort, makes you comfortable?

4. What/who are you attached to, connected to?

VIPS: Social

The final element of the VIPS is the social dimension of the person with dementia. Traditionally we believed the person living with dementia had no need for social interaction, as they were largely incapable of participating in or enjoying it.

This has been shown to be false in the modern care of people with dementia. The provision of opportunity to socialise for people living with dementia has shown that they can maintain their social capacity well into the progress of their disease, and indeed beyond the decline of verbal skills. Generally, the need to engage socially with others remains, despite decline in the ability to engage through verbal language. The desire to communicate, to attach, connect, be intimate, belong and feel 'like my old self' is sometimes as strong as it has ever been. It is perhaps *more* important, now that verbal language is not available and the person with dementia is reliant on others being sensitive to their nonverbal efforts to communicate their needs. Our social nature and innate desire for relationship is sustained even in the face of declining cognitive ability.

Some suggest that when words are lost we return to the pre-verbal way of relating to the world through feelings. This may be so. It makes emotional attachments formed in the pre-verbal period of life so much more important for our understanding of the motives and perspective of the person, and their needs for attachment, bonding and reliable presence from us. Essentially we have become attachment figures for them. We stand in the place of the early attachment figures who provided them with food, safety and affection in their pre-verbal life. So we may have emotional significance for them that extends far beyond what we ourselves are actually doing and may be more connected to the meaning of past attachment experiences for them.

In residential care or your own home, the person who lives with dementia needs social interaction that is consistent with their previous social preferences and current capacities. As we will see in Chapter 3, the changing effects of the dementia will affect the way the person is able to communicate socially. They may have diminished concentration or memory span, or word-finding difficulty. However, the *desire* to interact is often as strong as ever. As humans we are born in relationship with a 'mother' (who may or may not be our biological mother, and some people may have been nurtured as a young baby by their father), and then sustained in a network of relationships that provide physical nourishment, love and safety. This fosters the capacity for attachment and provides a secure base for movement out into the world of relationships, for exploration and adventure.

As a young person grows they develop self-esteem and a sense of themselves as loved and valued (or not). The sense of being loved may be conditional and the growing person comes to know that they are loved, so long as… Acceptance by others can be conditional upon them behaving in a pleasing manner, or doing good things, or not being angry, or… The list is endless.

In time people grow into adulthood and form attachments and create their own networks of love and friendship that support them into their adult years. Our sense of personal identity emerges from these attachments as we come to understand ourselves over the years.

These early experiences can shape the adult style of attachment. The person may have an anxious or ambivalent attachment style that shapes their personality and identity as they grow into adulthood. They may unconsciously shape themselves to conform to the emotional requirements of the other person – accepted and valued so long as they behave in a way that makes the other person happy with them. In popular psychology books this personal style may be known as a 'pleaser'. Much of their behaviour is designed to avoid rejection and be liked. If this is the major motive in their relationships, they will become very anxious and dependent if the person they are in relationship with begins to 'reject' them in the course of their dementia.

The adult may also adopt an avoidant style of relating and shun close relationships, keep to themselves, devalue closeness or intimacy or adopt an overly cognitive approach to relating. In dementia this may continue and manifest in unease with being close, or irritability with the dependence on others that their cognitive difficulties imposes on them.

Living with dementia, a person's attachment style remains fairly consistent with their previous pattern of relating with others. However, with the cognitive changes and uncertainty that often affect a person's social confidence when they begin making social mistakes, the attachment style can change. Often we see a reversion to previous attachment behaviour that may have been more common in the person's childhood or youth, such as clinging, dependency, insecurity or anxious/avoidant behaviour. As noted above, this can be a way of avoiding rejection by a loved one. Or it can be an attempt to regain control of an 'out-of-control' situation.

Such a reversion to previous styles of attachment can be seen as an attempt by the person to manipulate or control the carer. It is more likely, however, to be an attempt to preserve personhood in the simplest way they can. Rarely is the person able to sustain a complex strategy of social control such as manipulation!

And this is important to remember. A person you are caring for, in most circumstances, is not acting in a certain way just deliberately to annoy you. Even though their behaviour may cause an emotional reaction in you, just because you feel angry doesn't mean they are trying to make you angry or frustrate you. Don't interpret their behaviour in terms of how you feel about it.

So, bearing in mind this brief exploration of the social consequences of the person-centred way, and maintaining our focus on the well-being of the person we are communicating with, we will look in the next chapter at specific ways of communicating.

Exercise 2.4

VIPS – Social

1. What is your preference for social contact with others? A lot or a little?

2. Do others need permission to call on you or do you like spontaneous visits?

3. What do you like to have choice about?

4. In the past, have others treated you in such a way that you felt badly about yourself? If so, what did you do to protect yourself?

5. What is your attachment style? How does this influence you in your relationships?

6. What is the attachment style of someone you care for? How does it influence their behaviour? How can you act to help create well-being for them?

Chapter 3

How Do We Actually Communicate?

Communicating consists of listening and speaking. It also comprises emotions, perceptions and the many nonverbal aspects of interacting that help us understand each other and get our own message across to others.

Empathy, imagination and defensiveness

Before we consider the verbal and nonverbal components of communication it is important to consider empathy, imagination and defensiveness.

Empathy is simply defined as the capacity to understand another person's experience. It is a building block of communication. Without it there is no understanding, no common or shared perception of the situation. Empathy requires you to leave your own perspective temporarily and use your imagination to see and feel what it is like from the other person's point of view. Empathy and imagination go hand in hand. You need imagination to have empathy, to imagine life from someone else's frame of reference. What is it like to have dementia – to misunderstand, to make mistakes in conversation that you have not made before? What is it like to forget things you know you should know?

Not to be able to solve a problem that you know is simple, but you just can't do it today? Not to be able to dress yourself, because you can't remember the order of clothing? To become confused about what is going on? To lose track of a conversation and feel like you don't belong any more? What is it like to feel frightened because of this? Lonely? Isolated? Angry? Sad?

To communicate well with another person whose brain is changing, and not functioning the way it used to, requires imagination and empathy. To do it well you must bring your own feelings into the room as well. This may mean feeling things you might not be comfortable feeling. You might also be thinking things about the person that make you uncomfortable, such as 'I just wish they would go away.' Many caregivers think they must be unemotional or only feel good about their caring. This, however, leaves them at risk of being unable to empathise or understand the point of view and experience of the person they are caring for. To care in a person-centred way means bringing your whole self into the relationship, positive and negative feelings and all. Bring your emotions into the room.

Of course you must maintain your boundaries and remember that you have your own perspective, which is different from that of the person with dementia. But it is necessary to have a healthy engagement of your emotions in the person-centred way of caregiving.

We use empathy and imagination to communicate as we try to understand the experience of the other party. This is true at an international level when governments negotiate agreements such as trade deals. What is the other person/group saying and what do they mean?

What are their interests and motivations and how do we feel and think about this? What does it mean for me/my people? When there is understanding of what is driving each party and what is important to them, then there can be agreement and a way forward.

On an individual level we use empathy and imagination to try to understand each other in our marriages and intimate partnerships. When we lack empathy we create misunderstanding, and hurt results. Couple therapy sessions are full of individuals lacking empathy for the other person's experience. Only with imagination can they begin to see life from the other person's point of view. It is empathy when we can identify the feelings that go with that point of view.

The example of couple therapy allows us to see another interesting dimension of communication. And that is defensiveness. If you are feeling defensive and angry, afraid or sad, you may have difficulty having empathy for the other person. This is true in marital problems and other interpersonal difficulties, and it is true in caregiving. Your defensiveness may get in the way and prevent you being understanding and empathic about the experience of the person with dementia.

Defensiveness causes many problems in caregiving. In a close personal relationship with lots of history there may well be some defensiveness that has built up over the years. There may be good reason for it if your spouse has been difficult to live with, or domineering or dependent. Either way you will have a reaction to that behaviour that may have become a habitual defence against the difficult feelings it causes in you. In caregiving, then, when your spousal relationship changes from that status quo to a more fluid and unpredictable situation, you may find you have all sorts of feelings that concern you, and that you really do not want to feel or think about.

If this is happening it is recommended that you discuss these feelings with a professional counsellor who can help you understand them and find ways to manage them so that you can maintain your empathy and care for the person you are caring for. It is difficult to do it on your own because these feelings also have thoughts attached to them, and these thoughts can get in the way if they are negative or critical about the person you are caring for. It is very difficult to be objective about yourself and the other person when you are feeling defensive or have strong negative feelings.

So empathy and imagination are the building blocks of good communication in the person-centred way. Now we will build on them with verbal and nonverbal communication.

Verbal communication

Communicating in ordinary circumstances is composed traditionally of verbal and nonverbal parts. The verbal aspect is the words we use. This is thought to contribute only a small part of the overall meaning of what we communicate; figures vary from 5 to 30 per cent.

On the other hand, nonverbal cues are thought to contribute the major part of our communication, with estimates varying from 70 to 95 per cent. Nonverbal communication consists of body language and facial expression, as well as tone of voice, pitch, pace, and volume of sounds.

Words must be simple and direct. Use the KISS principle: 'Keep It Short and Simple'. As we have discussed in the earlier section 'Dementia and the Brain' (pages 12–19) the person may have decreased memory span and may also experience decreased ability to concentrate. So this means that sentences should be kept reasonably short and simple (but not childish). Generally you would avoid multiple phrases such as:

> The bus will be here at 10 o'clock and we'll go to the shops and get some fruit and veggies and then we can go to have coffee if you like. Would you like that?

(It may be that the person you are relating with *is* able to comprehend this sentence, in which case you could use it.)

Remember 'one size' does not fit all. Read their response. Are they confused or puzzled, or don't do what you have asked them to do? If so, change the way you speak. Do they smile, nod, respond with an appropriate comment? If so, you have hit the mark.

Judge what is appropriate by whether your speech meets with confusion or comprehension. Does it enhance or detract from the person's well-being? You can tell by referring to the list of signs of well-being and ill-being in the Appendix. It comes back to the basic rule: *avoid a one-size-fits-all approach to the care of people with dementia.* Adapt your speech to the person you are talking to with the aim of enhancing or sustaining their well-being as you go.

A point to remember: be careful to avoid simplistic sentences that might be interpreted by the person as 'baby talk'. You are still talking to an adult. Treat the person with respect and dignity.

Problems occur mostly when we fail to remember that the person has memory problems! Maybe we both have the problem.

Be specific

Say 'Put your hand on the rail' rather than 'Put your hand here'. As cognitive impairment progresses, the person may lose the words for some things and need your prompting. In the early period it is likely they will lose the connecting words in speech such as 'here' or 'there' and 'this' or 'that'. So when you speak, be specific about what you want them to do or not do. Below are some examples to help you find your own words for situations you are dealing with.

Vague	Specific
Put it over there.	Put the plate on the table.
Sit down.	Bend your knees. Put your bottom on the chair.
Give it to me.	Would you pass me the scissors, please?
Help me.	Take the bag in your hand.
Eat up.	Pick up your fork. Put it into the potato. Lift it to your mouth.
Walk with me.	Left foot. Now your right. Two steps.

One or two things at a time

As the person progresses in their dementia they may become less able to do complex (multi-step) activities like getting dressed or eating a meal without assistance. This may result in their being unable to follow a vague instruction such as 'Just get dressed and I will be back in a minute.' Getting dressed is too complex an idea. Break it up into the parts of dressing – for example, one step for each item of clothing or movement: 'Put your underpants on', 'Lift your foot', 'Put your arm in the sleeve. Now this arm' (touching the arm and holding the shirt sleeve open). You might place their clothes in the right order on the bed if they have difficulty with sequencing the series of actions but are able to dress themselves from that point.

Keep it short

As dementia progresses, the span of attention diminishes. The person may be unable to hold as much in their mind, for as long, as you and I can. When we are ill or tired our attention span also decreases, resulting in forgetting. 'Where did I put that..?'

The person may have trouble understanding or saying long sentences. So make your statements short and to the point. Avoid double-barrelled statements with 'and' in the middle. We are used to doing it in our conversation, but it can be confusing for people with a reduced attention span.

Consider the following examples:

Too long	Just right
Go over to the table and pick up the books and bring them over to me.	Go over to the table... Pick up the books... Bring them over to me.
Today we are going for a walk. Then we'll come back and have a game of bingo before tea. If we can, we might even go down the street for a coffee.	Today we are going for a walk. [Wait for acknowledgement that the person has understood you and then say the next idea] ... Then we'll have a game of bingo.

As well as being conscious of your own verbal communication, watch and listen for the person's verbal communication to you. How fluent are they? Are they able to complete a sentence? Do they need (or want) help finding words? Is the person forgetting the names of things? Remember, read their responses.

Always give your assistance with an eye on the person's emotional well-being. Look for the signs of well-being and ill-being. Think about how they are seeing the situation or task, and adapt your approach so that they can be successful. Hold back if you think offering help would only make it worse. Sometimes the best thing you can do is to remain silent and let the person find their own way out of the conversational (word-finding) situation they are in.

When breaking actions down doesn't help

It may be that the person you are caring for is unable to respond to your prompts to do an action because a stroke or the progress of the disease makes it impossible for them without your physical assistance. This is one of the most risky periods for the personhood of someone with dementia, because they are now more fully dependent on you and your insight, your skills, your empathy, your ability to adjust yourself to their needs and preferences, than ever before. They are much more at risk of being overwhelmed by generous but misguided caregivers who take over and 'do for' rather than 'do with'. Even in this condition of dependence you should be aiming to 'do with' the person, rather than for the person.

'Doing with' is not so easy when the person with dementia has limited verbal or cognitive ability to engage in the interaction as an equal participant. It is dependent upon our sensitivity and continued monitoring of their facial and gestural feedback to us. In such an interaction we must become astute 'readers' of their changing subtle signs of willingness to cooperate and participate, and signs of distress and refusal. Do you know what the signs of refusal are for the people you care for? They will vary from person to person. Some vocalise by calling out, groaning, screaming or shouting for help. Others will use more primitive behaviours to protect themselves from perceived harm and hit out, pinch, punch, kick or spit at you. These are strong signs of refusal and should be respected, first by making yourself and the other person safe, and then by moving away until the person no longer sees you as a threat.

'Doing with' is important here because it keeps you working alongside the person, rather than in opposition to them or with your own care agenda that may be unrelated to their mental and emotional perspective at the time. Just because they have dementia does not mean they cannot tell you what they want, prefer, desire. It keeps you looking for the cues that help you to empathise and understand their perspective. What are they feeling right now? Why might they be feeling that? Could it be their background? Could it be their past trauma and times of feeling trapped and overpowered that are making them think you are trying to do the same thing?

In this way, even though you as the caregiver are the one doing the care action for them, you are remaining connected to their mental and emotional state as much as possible. In this way you are 'doing with' the person.

Announcements

In what is commonly called an 'announcement' of care, you say what you are going to do prior to doing it (and avoid saying it *as* you are doing it), so that the person has plenty of notice that the care action is about to happen and can respond in some way, For example, the person you are caring for might benefit from having their position in a chair changed regularly, or require your help to go to the toilet, but they might be unable to request it or initiate it or cooperate with your instructions. They may be unable to contribute, and therefore be reliant on you doing the action for them.

There is a tendency for busy carers to work quickly when this occurs and to begin 'operating on' the person as if they were unconscious or an object. When people are not longer able to communicate verbally or contribute to their own self-care, we may fall into the trap of treating them in an impersonal manner. Just because they are old or have dementia does not mean they have no perspective on their care.

There is a high risk of this when caregivers are using equipment such a wheelchairs, lifting machines, blood sugar monitors, thermometers or blood pressure cuffs. All this equipment is helpful and at times necessary. However, with it comes a risk, and that is the risk of depersonalising the person we are helping.

Remember this person is a feeling being, a person who is reacting to, and having feelings about, what you are doing. If you have ever been carried in a lifting machine, you know how uncomfortable and frightening it can be to be swinging in mid-air, particularly if the people operating it are not focusing on your feelings and helping you to feel safe and cared for.

The announcement of care would sound like this:

Mrs Davis, hello, it's been an hour since we last moved you. I would like to move you again so you can be comfortable. Would that be OK?

The carer then waits for a sign of verbal or nonverbal agreement from Mrs Davis that she is willing to participate in this care action. Take this step slowly, so that the person has enough time to grasp what you are saying. Use a clear voice and be brief and to the point. Then wait for a response.

Jane is with me. We're going to sit you up and put a belt around you to...

All the time you are smiling and communicating calm and confidence in a slowly managed process. Do not move quickly or talk loudly (unless the person has hearing problems, of course). Keep up your conversation so that Mrs Davis knows what you are up to.

Once she has responded (if she can), or you have established that she cannot communicate her agreement, you proceed with moving her as gently, safely and quickly as possible.

You should watch her face and body for signs of distress, pain, worry, agitation, etc. If you see any of these signs, stop and reassess whether to proceed, or delay the care action, or not do it at all.

There are times when the risk of causing upset and distress outweighs the benefit of carrying out the care action, and then it is better not to do it until such time as the person is more agreeable or you can find another way to achieve your care goal. (If this happens in a workplace such as a nursing home or hostel you should always communicate what has happened to your manager so that documentation can be maintained about what has happened, and why.)

Announcing care actions is an important part of caring for someone with a progressively worsening condition like dementia. A person may be able to respond well and take up your prompts for a while, but then as the disease progresses they may become unable to do it, or at least unable to do it every time. You must be sensitive to the changes in the person's abilities and remember that their emotions are still active as their skills decline. They may well be angry about losing abilities they previously prided themselves on. This may be particularly true for males, who may be more inclined to be angry about loss of independence.

Remember to keep high the quality of your nonverbal interaction at this time. Don't move too fast, or be so focused on your task that you lose focus on the emotional and physical well-being of the person you have in your arms. Smile. Communicate on the same level as the person, rather than standing over them. They might have lost comprehension of your words, but they may still be perceiving your nonverbal communication. They will certainly be reacting to your physical care, so make it gentle, confident and calm. They need to feel your confidence in your ability to lift, hold and lead them in a way that lets them feel safe and remain calm.

For a discussion of relating with people without words or mobility, see Chapter 4.

Exercise 3.1

Communicating verbally

1. When have you had problems communicating with a person with dementia?

2. How did you deal with it? Was your response successful?

3. Give two examples of specific speech to a person with dementia.

4. Why should you keep instructions simple?

5. What length of instruction can the person you care for take in and deal with successfully?

6. When should you announce care actions? What is important to remember when using announcements rather than prompts?

Nonverbal communication

Nonverbal communication is by means of body language, tone, pitch and pace.

Let us look first at your body language. Body language is posture, facial expression, eye contact and gesture, i.e., how you use your body. Body language is a means of communicating, and 'body messages' can tell us a great deal if we take the time to watch and listen.

Smile

Your face is your best communicator. You can tell the other person so much about how you feel, and your feelings about them, by the way you smile. It tells them they are accepted and it's OK. It includes them. This keeps them in connection with you, listening and open to you. On the other hand, a frown sends a different message. Our focus is sustaining and building well-being, so obviously, the more you smile and have a relaxed face, the more likely it is that the other person will be positive and relaxed too. So smile, smile, smile!

Stand in front of the person when talking to them. Nonverbal communication is the most important aspect of communicating with people with progressing dementia. They rely on it more and more. So being able to see you, watch your face and other body messages is vital to helping them make sense of you and your message to them.

Eye contact is important as well. It has been said that the eyes are the window to the soul. Don't stare, but maintain an interested gaze for short periods. (Some cultures see this as inappropriate and rude, so match your approach to the perceptions and expectations of the person you are relating with. Again, avoid a 'one-size-fits-all' approach to communication.)

The person may have reduced memory and be easily distracted by noise. They may also have trouble concentrating on your voice or picking out your voice from a noisy background. (This is called 'figure-ground' and it applies to vision as well.) To maximise the chance of communicating successfully, make sure the person is looking at you. This way the person is more likely to hear your voice and see your mouth moving as channels of communication and be able to focus on it.

Posture

Your posture can tell the person whether you are interested in them or not. Lying back on the bed when visiting a person in their room will not encourage the person with dementia to keep talking to you as much as if you lean forward and look at them.

Gestures

Gestures can also be valuable, particularly if the person has lost much of their verbal communication ability. Use the visual channel to get your message across to them by means of actions that demonstrate what you want to tell them. Again, remember that certain gestures may be culturally offensive.

Tone of voice

In addition to body language, tone and pitch can change the meaning of what you say. We know that nonverbal cues are important in successful communication. This is even more important when talking with people who have dementia. Tone of voice, posture, gestures and facial expression will all send a signal to the person that either matches your words or not. As someone's ability to make sense of words decreases, their reliance on nonverbal parts of your communication will be more profound. So if you wish to have a positive relationship with the person, get your ideas across successfully and have them understood, then you must become more sensitive regarding your use of nonverbal cues and their effect on communication.

Use a tone that signals equality rather than 'I'm the boss'. The more the person feels equal, the more they will want to remain participating in your relationship. Their self-esteem is likely to be fragile as a result of feeling that they are failing at things, so make every effort to use a tone that tells them they are equal.

If you are not sure about your tone, ask for feedback from someone you trust: 'How do I sound when I talk to Tom? Does it sound like I am treating him as an equal or am I sounding patronising?'

Avoid telling the person off for mistakes they make: 'Tom, you've done it again. I told you yesterday not to eat like that.' No one likes to have their mistakes pointed out to them. They are most likely aware that they have made mistakes, and even if they are not, what good does it do to point it out repeatedly? Memory loss will rob the person of any good effect you are trying to achieve by reminding them of their mistake. All it leaves them with is a bad feeling about themselves and a desire not to have anything to do with you. Move on and continue speaking evenly and calmly to the person.

Christine was irritated by her husband, Ted, who had dementia and was forgetting things. She came home at the end of the day from work and found that he had pulled out old furniture from the garage and left it out on the lawn. He had mistakenly locked the dog in the tool shed and put the forks and spoons away in the wrong place in the kitchen. At first she became so annoyed that she corrected him each time, pointing out what he had done and how annoyed she was by it. He became defensive and at first denied he had been the one to lock the dog in the shed. It must have been someone else. He defended himself from what felt like an attack on his self-esteem. He withdrew and refused to talk. Christine was annoyed with him, and with herself for letting it get to her, and with his dementia, which she was struggling to cope with at times. She just wished he was the old Ted. She really missed him.

If a person's comprehension ability is impaired, it is vital to be clear and unambiguous about how you say things. An instruction such as 'Sit down and I will be back in a minute' can be delivered in a gentle tone, with kindness, or it may be delivered in a bullying way that really means, 'I will be very angry if you move before I get back'. This is a form of intimidation and should be avoided. Once again, be clear that you are communicating acceptance and encouragement.

Rate of speech

Let them chew it over... Speak at a rate that is acceptable and comprehensible to the person. Many of us speak quickly, and this can be a problem for the older person, whether they have dementia or not. Remember, don't shout. Because people live with dementia does not mean that they are deaf (although, of course, they may have a specific hearing impairment!).

As well as having a reduced attention span, the person with dementia may also find that they are not thinking or reacting as quickly as they used to. This happens naturally to us all as we age, but it is more pronounced in people living with dementia. If this happens you may find yourself hurrying the person without realising that they are not staying with you – in other words, you lost them some time ago.

Pauses

So, pause between ideas to give the person time to take in and make sense of what you are saying. This way you will find out how much they can actually process and make sense of. If you do not pause, all you will see is how confused the person becomes when faced with too much information. It is as if their mind gets indigestion. Give them time to chew it over before the next 'mind-full'.

This can be combined with breaking ideas down into short sentences and/or by introducing a brief pause between short sentences to support their comprehension.

How long should the pause be? About the time it takes you to say, 'One, one thousand'. It will vary from person to person, but if you begin here and adjust your timing to the person you are talking with, you will find an effective pause time that works for both of you. It may also vary with how tired or unwell the person is.

James and Alice had been married for 53 years when she began to be more forgetful than usual, and over the next few years James picked up more and more for her in conversation, so that if they were out together and he noticed she was faltering in a conversation he would seamlessly step alongside her and fill in the gaps. She felt good having him there, and together they were able to maintain their social life. At home Alice forgot what was happening next and would frequently stand alongside James and ask what he was doing. He patiently told her again, and she smiled as if hearing it for the first time.

Equality

Much communication with older people happens while they are sitting in a chair or wheelchair. If you are standing, this creates an unequal social interaction. It often results in people not listening or turning off from the conversation early if they feel overwhelmed or undervalued. In order to ensure they are treated with respect and maximise your chance of being listened to, place yourself at their height to maintain social equality, i.e., if they are sitting, get down to their height on your knees if possible. This way they are freer to make a choice rather than feeling compelled to 'obey' because of your seemingly authoritarian posture in relation to them.

The carer stood over him with a spoon poised before his face like a helicopter waiting to dive into his mouth. He knew he had to cooperate because she was always telling people off for not eating fast enough or making a mess with their food. She looked around and gave instructions to the other carers like a general giving orders. You always did as you were told when she was on.

The person's self-esteem may be fragile, especially if they are feeling that they are failing at things, so make every effort to use a tone that tells them they are equal in the relationship and have equal power, and are accepted and part of the flow of life.

Exercise 3.2

Communicating nonverbally

1. Find an example of a statement that can be said using two different tones of voice with entirely different meanings.

2. What nonverbal communication would you use to convey interest and attention?

3. How do you show that you are listening?

4. How would you use nonverbal communication to indicate that you are not a threat?

Chapter 4

Relating to People without Speech or Mobility

Dementia is a progressively advancing condition that gradually decreases the range of normal brain function so that in the advanced or 'end-stage', as it is sometimes called, the person may lose mobility and language. These are critical human abilities and losing them can rob us of the opportunity to experience well-being in overt, obvious ways. However, this does not have to be the case. It just makes it harder for the person with dementia to experience well-being. It also makes it more difficult for the partner or carer, as it places more responsibility on that person for providing opportunities, or ensuring that opportunities are provided, for the person with dementia to take up or experience.

> The carer wheeled the large, comfortable 'fall-out' chair to a position by the window so that Julie, who had quite advanced dementia, could look out and enjoy the sun and the plants outside. Nearby, fellow residents were engaged in a group activity at the table. There was much laughter and enjoyment. Despite the stiffness of her rigid body and the angle of the chair, she craned her head around to look at the

gathering nearby and remained like that for several minutes, joining in. Her desire for social connection, to be included, was alive and well.

Julie is a social being, a person who has a history, a sense of herself and desires. We remain social beings despite losing language and the ability to move about to engage in social interaction. When dementia has robbed a person of the ability to speak words fluently or tell us about their experience, the urge to be in relationship continues. Our emotions are not impaired by dementia, just our ability to meet our desires, wants and needs.

We see this most dramatically in the small eye movements and head-turning as someone tracks your movements across a room. They follow you, watching your every move. They move their body as they anticipate the pleasure of your presence, and crane their neck to become involved.

In these small signs we can recognise the desire for connection with us. Unfortunately many carers miss these micro-communications and act as though they think the person has already stopped wanting to communicate. *The desire to communicate does not die with the words.*

Once a carer thinks this way, you can see the change in their behaviour toward the person they are caring. They become less engaged and responsive, more task-focused and matter-of-fact about their work. They stop looking at the person's eyes and face. They just do the work necessary to keep the person clean and fed.

This adds to the sense of disconnection, isolation and diminishing of personhood that is felt by the person being cared for.

For some family members who visit, or who care for a relative at home, this is the only way they are able to relate with the person – because it can be too painful to know they are still here but changed, too painful altogether. So they split off from their relative as if they have gone and are no longer present. It's safer emotionally.

We can be compassionate towards families who react in this way. It is rarely out of malice that they treat the person with dementia badly. Mostly it is the best they can manage. What we can do is model for them how to include their family member in conversation by speaking to them, referring to them as we talk and never ignoring them in conversation.

Perhaps the most difficult situation for many carers occurs when the person they care for has become so disabled by the effects of the disease process that they seem able only to experience sensory life, are reliant on us for all their activities of daily life and are unable to communicate using words.

Even if we cannot see the eye movements or other signs of recognition, *the person with dementia is still in relationship with us, and we with them.*

Personhood remains as long as the person has breath. It is sometimes extremely difficult to see or sense the person in this physically changed state, lying in a chair or in bed, unable to speak or take care of themselves.

Communication is still two-way, however, and we need eyes to see it. John Killick is a man who can see it. He has written beautifully about the poems that people with dementia have produced, revealing their perceptions of the world, themselves and their lives. These poems by people with dementia can be found in two volumes: *You are Words: Dementia Poems* (Killick 1997) and *Openings* (Killick and Cordonnier 2000).[1]

These very important poems have opened up and confirmed for us that people in the advanced stages of dementia retain a sense of themselves, the world and their own life. They want to remain in connection with the people they love, and who love them.

The person may use micro-behaviours such as eye movements, facial expressions, head movements, small gestures, vocalising and silences to tell us what they are experiencing, or want or need. These small signs of relating to the external world are messages that hold meaning. They are the person's language in this stage of the journey. This language is small and quiet and requires understanding born in silence and waiting. It is in this quiet space that the memories of who they are, and were, remain our connecting points and stimulate us to keep them in the forefront of our minds: a person in all their richness, whose past becomes present in our thoughts.

During this period of being with a person with dementia who is unable to speak or care for themselves, we are charged with holding their personhood in our hands. We do this in our memories of them, our stories about them and in our gentle and thoughtful attempts to offer them comfort, sustain attachment, affirm identity,

1   John Killick also has a website: www.dementiapositive.co.uk.

engage in occupation and meet their entitlement to inclusion as a person among equals.

Managing your own needs

We must manage our own neediness at this time. Emotionally this is a draining time that can be very difficult and cause many people to move away from someone with dementia. It can be confronting to sit with, or bathe or clean a person who is in such a dependent state of being. It confronts us with our own mortality and past or present youth, our own desire for speed and results. We must manage this distress. It is rarely possible on our own. This is a time to connect with those who love us and can help sustain us with their support and often practical encouragement.

This challenging and difficult time has the potential to be a profoundly growing time for those around the person with dementia, whether you are a paid carer or family carer. You will discover things about yourself that you did not know, things you like and things you do not like about yourself. This is part of the experience of caring, and one to be embraced and respected. If you have the opportunity, seek out someone to talk this through with, so that you can learn and grow from it.

Exercise 4.1

Relating to people without words or mobility

1. What micro-behaviours are important to notice when communicating with someone who has lost the power of speech?

2. How can you improve the experience of someone who has lost words?

3. What nonverbal communication is useful when communicating with someone who has lost words?

Chapter 5

Specific Situations

I would say, 'You know what, Helen? I know your
daughter, and I talked with her today about you. She
told me that you grew up in Chippewa Falls and that
you were living on a farm. Do you remember that
place?' As these personal prompts helped [her] to
connect and retrieve from memory, mentioning the
resident's daughter or son also enabled her to relate
to me as a 'friend', someone who could be trusted.

Habib Chaudhury (Chaudhury 2008, p.79)

Daily life for a person with dementia can be a challenge
that at times seems insurmountable. Good communication
during the activities of daily living (ADLs) can make
all the difference. We will look now at several everyday
activities that can be enhanced by good communication.

In the shower

When assisting someone with dementia in the shower it
is important to remember the nature of the situation you
are in. It is a very private space in the bathroom where
the person has probably never had someone else in
there with them. Showering is usually a solitary activity
that is extremely private. The person is naked or being
helped to undress by you.

In this situation, how are they likely to feel? This is the vital question, as it has been all the way through this book. How are they likely to feel? How would you feel?

It is reasonable to suppose that they may feel embarrassed, frightened, angry, or even just confused and perhaps then angry, or anxious and worried that something bad is going to happen to them.

Being naked in front of someone else is not something that many older people (actually, many people) have been (and remain) comfortable with, so we must offer the person understanding of their likely discomfort.

For many women, fear of sexual attack is common, and men may also experience fear related to the vulnerability of being naked. Remember that when someone feels like this they may act in a defensive or protective way to defend themselves from a possible threat or danger. Previous traumatic experience (such as surviving the Holocaust) can cause the person to act as if the traumatic event is occurring again in the present. This can be distressing for both the person with dementia and for the carer, who is doing their best to provide good care, only to be misunderstood by the person in distress.

In case of a traumatic or catastrophic response, first back off as far as it is safe to do so. (You may not be able to leave the person alone, due to safety concerns, but withdraw physically so that you do not pose a threat to the person.) Speak in a soft, calming voice and smile. Hold your hands palms out and fingers up, signalling 'no threat'. Give all the signals you can think of to demonstrate that there is no threat and only safety and security here.

Many carers are assaulted in the close confines of a shower space. So it is important to think it through before you enter such a potentially volatile situation. Always talk to the person with dementia so that they know what you are doing or what you are about to do. Give them plenty of notice and make sure you keep up the talk, to let them know all the time what you are doing. If you stop talking, they may forget what you are there for and become confused and angry/anxious/worried and terrified. So keep talking about anything – perhaps about the person and their life, if you know enough about them, or about yourself and your children, or what they are going to do today. As noted earlier, it is crucial to know the person's life-story so that you can stimulate feelings of well-being during times when they are under stress because of the illness.

If you know the person is concerned about their privacy, try at all times to keep them covered by a towel, so that they do not feel so exposed. Some people may actually prefer to shower in their night attire, and then you can remove it when convenient in the process of showering.

Use the physical environment to help maximise the likelihood of success. Lovely smells with aromatherapy, a warm bathroom, warm towels, a hot face-washer, soothing (or the person's favourite) music all increase the chance of positive feelings and a good outcome. Prepare, and you will benefit. So will the person!

Act relaxed and try to be relaxed. Give nonverbal signals of relaxation that the person can pick up and respond to accordingly. If they pick up that you are tense and on edge, you are likely to lose rapport and they may enter a defensive and protective mood in which it is more likely that angry feelings will be expressed.

Your demeanour must not be bossy. If you are in a hurry, or have the attitude that they must have a shower 'because I know what is best for you', you will have problems on your hands.

If this happens, step back and use humour if you can, to defuse and change the mood. A smile always works wonders, even if the last thing you feel like doing is smiling.

When a person is agitated and not cooperating, cease the showering, ensure that their body is covered, and change to something else – like a manual face-wash, by giving them a warm face-washer to hold and use.

A face-washer may also be useful to hand to the person if they are hitting out during showering, so that they have something to hold and are not grabbing onto you.

If the person is reluctant to enter the shower, you may benefit from turning on the water as you talk to them and gradually lead them to accept the shower – all the time maintaining their freedom to choose not to have one.

It is not necessary to give a full shower every day if the person's hygiene is good. This may alleviate stress for them. If they are incontinent, however, you may need to offer a full shower daily.

At mealtimes

Mealtimes are important times in the day when we not only consume food but can join others for conversation and sharing of experience and memories. This is a wonderful opportunity, in an aged care home or in a person's family home, to share experiences of reminiscence and closeness with others, as well as good food.

A meal can be enjoyable, or it can be a functional feeding time. You choose. How it is for the person with dementia is very much up to you as the able person in the interaction.

To understand what a meal can do for people, I suggest you watch a film entitled *Babette's Feast* (Axel 1987). In this tale, set in a small Danish village dominated by a religious conservatism that restricts enjoyment of even basic things like food, a meal of delicious dishes and fine wine, beautifully prepared by Babette, transforms the lives of those who sit around the table. They are freed to connect and enjoy like never before. They see each other as if for the first time. Memories are kindled, and loves emerge from the cold past.

Only give as much assistance as someone needs to eat their meal successfully. Sometimes this may be as little as a verbal prompt, and on other days it may start there and gradually increase, as it becomes obvious that they are having a bad day and need more help. Sit down at their level, facing the person, or to one side, so that you can use the fork or spoon straight on. Offer just enough food on the spoon or fork for the person to take it all in one mouthful. If you need to clean their face with a spoon or cloth, it may be that you presented too much food.

Try to assist only one person at a time, if you are in a communal setting. Give your attention to that person, and carry on a conversation as you would with anyone else at mealtime. Take your time, and help at their pace. Give them time to swallow, and always watch for finishing a mouthful. Watch for the swallow before you offer the next spoonful of food.

If the people you are with at mealtimes are able to converse, your presence can help them to maintain good social skills of conversation and eating in public, as they watch you eat or model their behaviour on yours. If you are eating at home, sit with the person with dementia so that they can see you eat, and model appropriate eating for them. You can do this when you eat out as well. This gives them confidence that they are eating appropriately. Sit opposite them so that they can see what you do. Eating may or may not be a problem, but if you do identify it as such, this may help. In communal settings some people may sit waiting until everyone is seated before they start eating. It is important to remember that many of the generation of people for whom we care were educated by their parents that it was bad manners to start eating until everybody at the table commenced.

Once the meal is underway, conversation can enhance eating it by stimulating the person's good feeling, helping them to relax and feel that they are in familiar surroundings with familiar people, who they feel good to be with. You can talk about familiar memories of events, people and foods that they like and enjoy, to help the person feel good. This contributes to well-being in a situation that could otherwise be a functional, barren experience that is frustrating for both parties.

Finger food

Talking together at mealtimes can be a problem if the person is not able to sit for an entire meal. So it may help to have a finger-food menu available so that the person can move about freely and still have nutrition. A finger-food menu may also be useful if the person is unable to use utensils any more. A broad range of food is possible in a finger-food format, from sandwiches to firm pieces of cooked vegetables (contact dieticans in your area for advice).

Dressing

How we dress communicates our identity to others. Making sure a person with dementia is dressed in a manner appropriate to their preferences, activity and identity is an important responsibility.

Helping a person to dress is a time for some lightness, and a preparation for the day ahead. Conversation here can be an important mood-setter. Think about what mood the person is in and what lies ahead for the day. You may want to help them move out of a dark or confused mood by focusing on a topic you know gives them pleasure. Keep your focus on them as a person, rather than just as someone you have to dress. Have the life-story book close by, so that you can open it at a prepared page and begin the conversation with a comment about an event from their past that you know gives them pleasure. Even if they cannot join in the talk, they will pick up your nonverbal interest and relaxed rapport and be more likely to enter the day in a positive mood.

Suggesting choices as the person dresses can be an important way to sustain well-being and build confidence to function in the world. By providing just enough assistance for them to succeed independently, you can set them up for a positive approach to the day. Make the choices simple and according to their ability, so as to produce a successful result: ask questions such as, 'Would you like to wear this dress, or this dress?' An even simpler choice would be, 'Would you like to wear this dress?'

Sometimes you may have to be assertive to guide the person in a direction that will lead to a good outcome. This must be done carefully, so that the person does not feel dominated. Watch skilful colleagues who are good at it. Learn from them. They know when to hold back and let the person go ahead, and when to step in and provide guidance in a particular direction in a way that preserves the person's dignity.

Going to the toilet

Helping someone maintain their continence is an important part of respect for their dignity. Social gaffes of wetting yourself in public can result in huge embarrassment and withdrawal. Remember that toileting is not just a matter of keeping to a two-hourly schedule. It is about remembering the value of this function to the person. Much self-esteem and personal dignity is tied up with the bodily functions of urinating and defecating.

So how we approach the person will have consequences for their well-being. Always speak quietly, if possible, when inviting someone to go to the toilet.

Always invite, rather than instruct or compel them to go to the toilet. Offer choice if possible. Make suggestions. Some staff think that a 'No' means they should back off and let it go, but there are other options at that point. Come back later, revisit the topic by making an observation that the person might be close to needing the toilet and you are there to help if they do – 'What about I help you now?' Always respect and preserve the person's right to refuse. Get permission before removing clothing. This is respectful, and sensible too. It is not worth keeping the person continent at the cost of their emotional well-being and creating bad feelings and a break of trust with you. A discreet change of clothes and a loving approach can always soothe a temporary loss of dignity or embarrassment. This is much to be preferred than your becoming associated in their mind with distress and incontinence.

Going out

Being in social situations such as shopping, at sporting events, the cinema or restaurants should all remain on the agenda for a person with dementia until such time as it becomes too stressful for them, or for you as their carer.

It is crucial that they be dressed appropriately for the event so that they do not stand out and attract negative attention, and are able to fit in with their usual social setting and group of peers. This is vital for their continued successful social participation and inclusion. It satisfies their need for belonging and identity and gives them an opportunity to feel beautiful and attractive, or professional, as appropriate for meeting each person's need to 'feel like my old self'.

Prepare for trips by assessing whether it is better to give plenty of notice or only a little notice. Some people become anxious if you tell them too far in advance about a trip to the shops, so perhaps tell them only 30 minutes beforehand, with time enough to prepare with a change of clothing. This may be different from how it used to be for them, but this is the way you must assess situations now – what works for them in the present and not what worked for them in the past. If this is going to work for both of you, it must be focused on the person's present needs rather than on what they used to prefer. This is often difficult for family caregivers. So if you care for your spouse or parent, you may need to adjust your thinking. That is quick and easy to say, and emotionally extremely difficult to do well. So be patient if you don't get it right or find it difficult to do consistently.

Getting bored

You and I can occupy ourselves successfully most of the time. A day of doing nothing sounds most attractive! The brain changes of dementia may mean that someone is unable to do the things that normally enabled them to be engaged and productive. This includes remembering tasks to do, starting by yourself, concentrating, sequencing, finishing, solving problems and thinking about the effect of our behaviour on others.

Inertia and lack of activity can result in disengagement, boredom and ultimately depression if allowed to go on for long enough. It is very difficult to re-engage someone once they have disengaged significantly, as the brain disease process will gradually rob them of the abilities they need to engage.

You may need to tailor the person's activity to what they can do and provide the support they need to fill in the gaps that dementia has created. This can mean offering opportunities according to their ability to succeed, and connected to their past, such that they can find meaning in an activity. Choose one that they find interesting, familiar and within their concentration span. Then be ready to provide the support necessary for success – and only that much. Do not take over.

Making mistakes

A lifestyle staff member gathered the group of residents for the craft activity and handed out the plaster ducks and birds for them to paint. All was ready, and the residents painted with enthusiasm until a volunteer stated loudly, 'Ducks aren't red, they're brown or white.' The person's face fell as she realised she had got it wrong.

Do not correct incorrect performance. Success is not measured by lack of mistakes but by participation and subjective feelings of success. Always focus on supporting the person in such a way that they have opportunity to experience well-being.

Pointing out mistakes in the actions or recollections of a person with dementia can have catastrophic effects on their well-being. This can be confronting for us in our own efforts to achieve accuracy. It's OK not to get it right, and the person with dementia can remind us of this very important truth.

Exercise 5.1

Specific situations

1. How can you maintain rapport when showering someone with dementia?

2. What is important to remember about assisting someone to eat?

3. How might you invite someone to go to the toilet if you know a refusal is likely?

4. Offering choices is important, so how would you help someone to get dressed if they need help with making choices?

Chapter 6

Caring for Yourself

Caring for another person can be a draining experience, as well as a most rewarding one. We can cope with the rewarding times! It's the difficult times that cause us distress and crises of confidence about ourselves, or moments of utter frustration with the situation.

When you have reached your limit

We each have a stress threshold below which we can feel OK, behave in a normal manner and cope well with challenges. Above this threshold we begin to feel overwhelmed and upset, and the normal everyday things that usually wouldn't bother us become annoying, difficult and stressful.

What is your limit? And how do you know when you have reached it? Each of us is slightly different in reading the signs of our own distress. When caring for someone else the stresses can be subtle and can increase over time without us realising it. Only on reaching the threshold do we notice the strain we have been under. What are your signs of stress?

What do you do when you have reached your limit and you are about to explode? Below are a few quick suggestions, to which you can add your own.

- Go for a walk.

- Physically move out of where you are.

- Phone a friend.

- Breathe slowly.

- Dig the garden.

- Remind yourself: it's the disease.

Staying away from your limit

Caring about yourself as a carer is as important as any of the direct caring actions you might do for the person themselves. In caring for yourself, you do the person a favour by making sure that you stay well and peaceful and able to focus on their needs when next you care for them.

There are 'four pillars' of good health that you can focus on when considering how to look after yourself.

1. Good friends

Keep up your social life as much as possible. This is particularly important for people caring for a family member at home. Social life can take second place, all the more if the person you care for has lost some of the social ability they once had. It can be easier to stay at home. Socialising keeps you stimulated and interested in a world beyond the the walls of your house. This will help to keep you positive and away from a depressive view of the world, yourself and the person you care for.

2. Good food

If you eat well, you will stay well and healthy. So will the person you care for. If you eat poorly due to lack of interest, you should contact your GP to ask him or her about depression. Lack of appetite can be a sign of depression and should be taken seriously, as this is a risk for carers who are socially isolated and tired from the caring work.

3. Good sleep

Rest is restorative. How much do you need to feel rested? If you are caring for a family member it can be very difficult to get good sleep, particularly if the person's own sleep pattern is disturbed. If you share a bed with them, this can be even more complicated.

Sleep has rhythm to it and you can prepare for sleep by taking time to slow your system down before going to be. Avoid things such as coffee and other stimulants, and avoid eating late in the evening. Establishing a good pre-sleep routine can help you and the person you care for.

For a professional carer good sleep is just as important, and easier to maintain. You will need to make sure you get good sleep before your shifts.

4. Good exercise

Caring for someone with dementia will ensure that you get good exercise, but you may need to ensure that you get out of the house for a walk with the person you care for, perhaps for the change of scene as much as for the exercise. Good blood flow to the brain is essential, and the 'feel-good' hormones that are released by vigorous exercise can lift our mood out of a low state.

With these 'four pillars' you will keep the building that is yourself in good condition to face the stresses and challenges of caring for a person with dementia.

Daily routine with space for your needs

A routine is valuable both for the person living with dementia and for you, if only to bring some predictability to a somewhat changeable situation. Each day should have a balance, within that routine, of time in active caring and time for you that is not involved in direct caregiving. This is important both for your own mental health and for the person you are caring for. You will be no help if you are exhausted or burned out.

This space for you can be as simple as regular time to rest with your eyes closed and your head back, focusing on pleasant memories of places or people. Sounds simple – but in the moment it can be rather difficult to maintain. The daily discipline of it is what makes it therapeutic.

Carers get depressed sometimes

We can all get 'down' and 'blue' or negative about our situation. This can develop into depression, and for some people this is an experience that plagues them throughout their lives. Carers are vulnerable to becoming depressed. Studies have shown that home-based carers have higher rates of depression than other people the same age. The social isolation of caring for someone in your own home and the draining daily constancy of it can be wearing. Also the loss of previously enjoyable activities can be saddening. To counter this effect it is crucial that the 'four pillars' described above become a focus for the home carer. It is helpful for us all to have this focus to prevent a slide into a depressed state.

What resources do you have?

No matter how isolated or withdrawn or overwhelmed by the demands of caring, each of us has some resources upon which to draw in times of need. It can be difficult to bring them to mind when you are in the midst of the needy situation, and it may be helpful to list the resources that you have so that you can bring them to mind when you need them. Categories of resources might include:

- Family I can rely on.

- Friends I can call on.

- Neighbours I can call on or visit.

- Interests/hobbies.

- Groups I belong to.

- Personal qualities I have.

- Affirming statements I can make to myself.

Caring for another person is a privilege and a joy most of the time. One of the most important human actions we can do for each other is to care for another person in their need. Caring for people who live with dementia is just such a privileged relationship.

Exercise 6.1

Caring for yourself

1. List the ways you recognise stress in yourself.

2. What personal qualities are helping you stay well, emotionally and physically?

3. List the ways you are looking after yourself under the Four Pillars:

    a. Good food

        i. What are you doing to ensure you eat well?

        ii. When was the last time you ate out with friends?

    b. Good friends

        i. How are you keeping up with friends?

        ii. When was the last time you phoned a friend and talked about yourself?

        iii. When did you last go out to see a film?

    c. Good sleep

        i. What is your sleep routine?

        ii. How many hours per night do you need to feel rested?

        iii. How many hours do you get?

        iv. How do you make sure you have a good night's sleep?

        v. What do you do when sleep is poor?

    d. Good exercise

       i. How often do you walk for 20–30 minutes?

      ii. When was your last physical check-up with a GP?

4. What resources do you have that you can call on if you need help?

5. How does your self-talk (comments you make to yourself) bring your mood down and how does it help you to keep going?

Conclusion

I hope the person-centred approach to caring helps you to communicate, relate well and have insight into the world of the people you care for. The world of dementia can be confusing and fearful at times, both for the person living with it and for those around them. As you enter the world of another person, your care and communication can help make their experience enjoyable, peaceful and dignified, and will enhance and sustain their personhood as you journey along using the person-centred approach through dementia with them.

Appendix

Signs of well-being

- Communicates wishes/needs successfully
- Engaged with the people, things and events around them
- Sensitive to the emotional needs of others
- Positive mood shown in smiling, laughing
- Engages in creative activity such as painting, singing, dancing
- Shows enjoyment in interactions and events
- Shows awareness of the well-being of others by being helpful
- Makes social contact (eye contact, begins conversation, touches others appropriately)
- Can be affectionate
- Shows self-respect in attention to dress and appearance
- Bodily relaxation (facial expression and body posture)
- Humour, playfulness

- Cooperative with requests
- Enjoys life
- Confident
- Cheerful
- Willingly participates in care
- Trusts others
- Comfortable with physical closeness

Signs of ill-being

- Negative mood (shows upset in facial expression, posture and sounds such as whimpering, calling out, screaming or crying)
- Walks into other people's private space or into unsafe areas
- Grieving, sad
- Angry, aggressive
- Agitated or restless
- Shows anxiety or fear
- Boredom
- Bodily tension
- Easily dominated by others
- Rejected or ignored by others
- Listlessness, apathy
- Withdrawal

- Physical discomfort or pain
- Unable to enjoy things
- Lonely
- Makes noise, calls out or vocalises
- Verbally refuses care
- Suspicious of others
- Physically threatens others

References

Axel, G. (1987) *Babette's Feast* (film).

Bradford Dementia Group (2005) *Dementia Care Mapping: Principles and Practice.* University of Bradford: Bradford Dementia Group.

Brooker, D. (2004) 'What is person-centred care in dementia?' *Reviews in Clinical Gerontology 13*, 1–8.

Brooker, D. (2007) *Person-centred Dementia Care: Making Services Better.* London: Jessica Kingsley Publishers.

Chaudhury, H. (2008) *Remembering Home: Rediscovering the Self in Dementia.* Baltimore, MD: The Johns Hopkins University Press.

Killick, J. (1997) *You Are Words: Dementia Poems.* London: Hawker.

Killick, J. and Cordonnier, C. (2000) *Openings: Dementia Poems and Photographs.* London: Hawker.

Kitwood, T. (1997) *Dementia Reconsidered: The Person Comes First.* Buckingham: Open University Press.

Kitwood, T. and Bredin, K. (1992) 'Towards a theory of dementia care: personhood and wellbeing.' *Ageing and Society 12*, 269–287.

Index